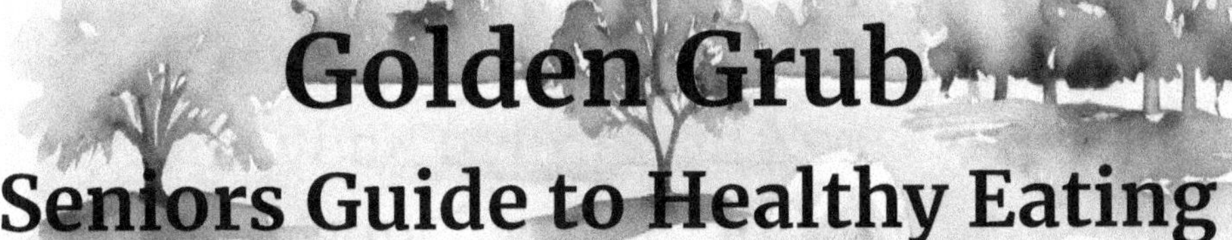

Golden Grub

Seniors Guide to Healthy Eating

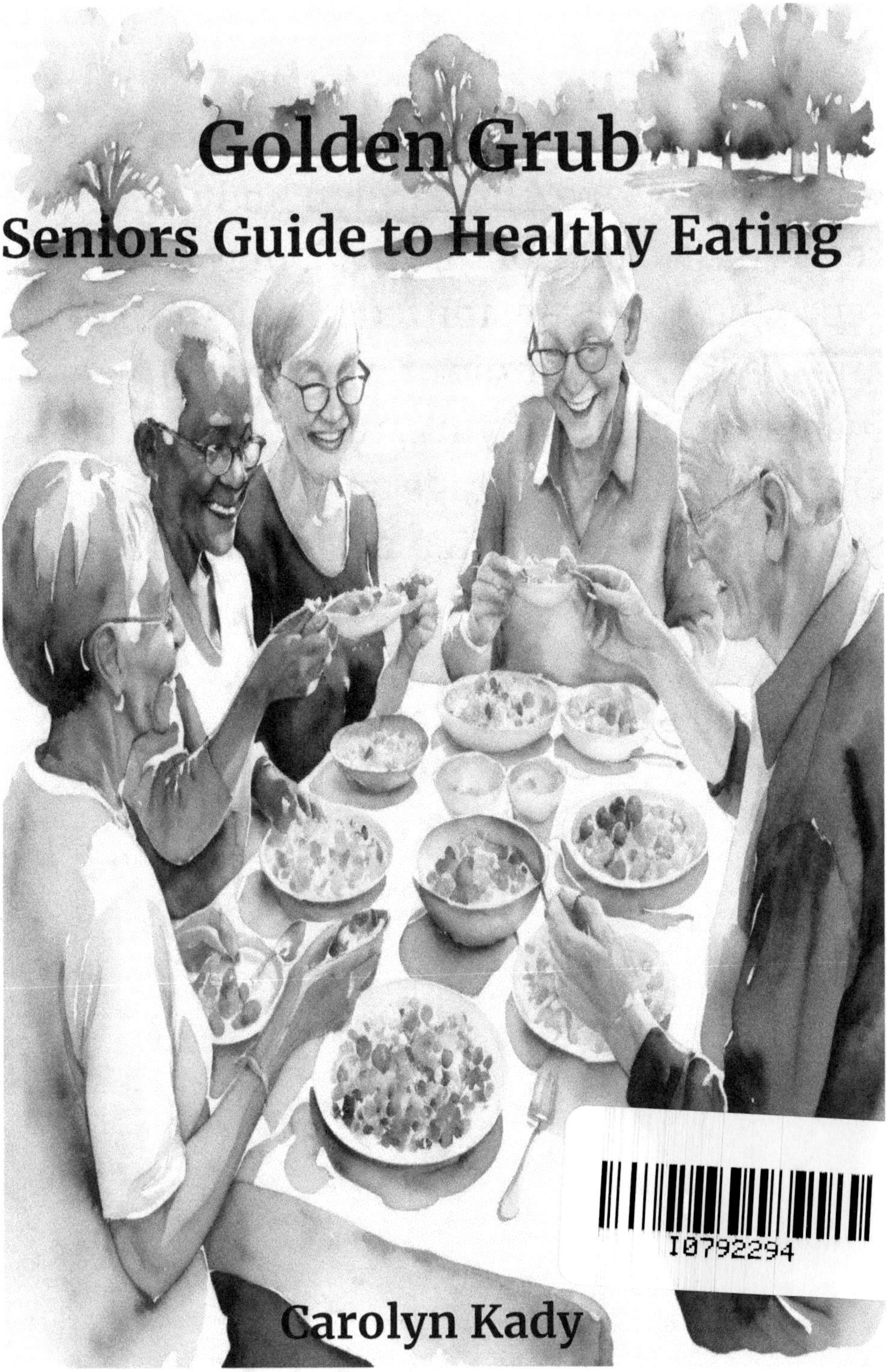

Carolyn Kady

DISCLAIMER

The information contained in this book is for general informational purposes only. It is not intended to provide legal, financial, or medical advice. The author of this book is not a licensed professional in any field and does not hold themselves out as such.

Table of Contents

Chapter 1: Introduction to Senior Nutrition

As individuals age, their nutritional needs change. Proper nutrition is crucial for seniors to maintain good health and well-being. In this chapter, we will explore the importance of nutrition for seniors and how it can improve overall health and quality of life.

As we age, our bodies undergo various physiological changes that can impact our ability to absorb nutrients. Seniors may also experience a decline in appetite, which can lead to malnutrition and other health issues. Additionally, certain medical conditions and medications can affect nutrient absorption and metabolism. This makes it essential for seniors to pay close attention to their diet and ensure they are meeting their nutritional needs.

Nutrition plays a critical role in maintaining overall health and well-being for seniors. A balanced diet provides essential nutrients that support the body's immune system, promote healthy aging, and reduce the risk of chronic diseases. Adequate intake of vitamins, minerals, protein, and fiber is essential for seniors to stay healthy and active.

Proper nutrition can also help seniors maintain a healthy weight, which is important for reducing the risk of obesity-related health problems such as diabetes, heart disease, and arthritis. Maintaining a healthy weight can also improve mobility and reduce the risk of falls and fractures.

In addition to physical health benefits, nutrition can also have a positive impact on mental health and cognitive function. A diet rich in antioxidants, omega-3 fatty acids, and other nutrients can help protect brain health and reduce the risk of cognitive decline and dementia. Good nutrition can also improve mood and overall quality of life for seniors.

It is important for seniors to consume a variety of foods from all food groups to ensure they are getting a wide range of nutrients. A balanced diet should include plenty of fruits and vegetables, whole grains, lean protein sources, and healthy fats. Seniors should also stay hydrated by drinking plenty of water throughout the day.

In addition to eating a balanced diet, seniors should also pay attention to portion sizes and meal timing. Eating smaller, more frequent meals throughout the day can help regulate blood sugar levels and prevent overeating. It is also important for seniors to avoid excessive salt, sugar, and processed foods, which can contribute to health problems such as high blood pressure, diabetes, and obesity.

In some cases, seniors may need to take dietary supplements to meet their nutritional needs. Vitamin D, calcium, and B vitamins are common supplements recommended for seniors to support bone health, energy levels, and cognitive function.

It is important for seniors to consult with a healthcare provider before taking any supplements to ensure they are safe and appropriate for their individual needs.

In conclusion, nutrition is a key component of overall health and well-being for seniors. A balanced diet that meets the individual nutritional needs of seniors can help prevent chronic diseases, maintain a healthy weight, and support brain health and cognitive function. By paying attention to their diet and making healthy food choices, seniors can improve their quality of life and enjoy a longer, healthier, and more active lifestyle.

Chapter 2: Key Nutrients for Seniors

As we age, our nutritional needs change, and it becomes increasingly important to pay attention to the essential nutrients that our bodies require for optimal health. In this chapter, we will take a detailed look at the key nutrients that seniors need to support their overall well-being, including vitamins, minerals, and fiber.

Vitamins play a crucial role in maintaining good health as we age. Vitamin D, for example, is essential for bone health and muscle function, both of which can decline with age. Many seniors are at risk for vitamin D deficiency, as our bodies become less efficient at producing this vitamin when exposed to sunlight.

To ensure adequate intake, seniors should include vitamin D-rich foods in their diet, such as fatty fish, fortified dairy products, and egg yolks, or consider taking a vitamin D supplement if recommended by their healthcare provider.

Another important vitamin for seniors is vitamin B12, which is necessary for proper nerve function and red blood cell production. As we age, our bodies may have difficulty absorbing vitamin B12 from food, leading to a deficiency that can cause symptoms such as fatigue, weakness, and cognitive impairment. Seniors can increase their intake of vitamin B12 by consuming animal products like meat, fish, and dairy, or by taking a vitamin B12 supplement if advised by a healthcare provider.

In addition to vitamins, minerals are also essential for senior health. Calcium is particularly important for maintaining strong bones and preventing osteoporosis, a common condition among older adults that can increase the risk of fractures. Seniors should aim to include calcium-rich foods in their diet, such as dairy products, leafy greens, and fortified foods, or consider taking a calcium supplement if needed to meet their daily requirements.

Another mineral that seniors should pay attention to is potassium, which helps regulate fluid balance, muscle contractions, and blood pressure. Many seniors do not consume enough potassium in their diet, which can increase the risk of high blood pressure and other cardiovascular issues.

Potassium-rich foods include bananas, potatoes, oranges, and spinach, so seniors should aim to incorporate these foods into their meals to support heart health.

In addition to vitamins and minerals, fiber is another key nutrient that seniors need for optimal health. Fiber helps promote regular bowel movements, prevent constipation, and lower the risk of chronic diseases such as heart disease and type 2 diabetes. Seniors should aim to increase their fiber intake by including whole grains, fruits, vegetables, and legumes in their diet, as well as staying hydrated to support proper digestion.

Overall, seniors should focus on consuming a balanced diet that includes a variety of nutrient-rich foods to support their overall health and well-being.

In addition to vitamins, minerals, and fiber, seniors should also pay attention to their protein intake to support muscle mass and strength, as well as stay hydrated to maintain proper hydration levels.

In the next chapter, we will discuss the importance of hydration for seniors and provide tips for staying properly hydrated as we age. By paying attention to these key nutrients and making small changes to our diet and lifestyle, seniors can support their health and vitality well into their golden years.

Chapter 3: Meal Planning for Seniors

As we age, our bodies undergo various changes that can affect our dietary needs and eating habits. It is essential for seniors to carefully plan their meals to ensure that they are getting the necessary nutrients to support their overall health and well-being. In this chapter, we will discuss tips and strategies for planning nutritious meals that meet the unique dietary needs of seniors.

Consult with a Healthcare Provider

Before embarking on any meal planning for seniors, it is important to consult with a healthcare provider or a registered dietitian. They can provide valuable guidance on specific dietary needs based on individual health conditions, medications, and lifestyle factors.

They can also help identify any potential nutrient deficiencies that need to be addressed in the meal plan.

Focus on Nutrient-Rich Foods

Seniors should aim to include a variety of nutrient-rich foods in their meals to ensure that they are getting all the essential vitamins and minerals. This includes fruits, vegetables, whole grains, lean proteins, and healthy fats. It is important to prioritize foods that are high in fiber, calcium, vitamin D, and B vitamins, as these are often lacking in the diets of seniors.

Plan Balanced Meals

When planning meals for seniors, it is important to focus on creating balanced meals that include a variety of food groups.

A good rule of thumb is to include a source of protein, such as lean meats, poultry, fish, eggs, or legumes, at each meal. Pair protein with whole grains, such as brown rice or quinoa, and plenty of colorful fruits and vegetables to create a well-rounded meal.

Adapt Recipes for Dietary Restrictions

Many seniors may have dietary restrictions due to health conditions such as diabetes, high blood pressure, or food allergies. When planning meals, it is important to adapt recipes to accommodate these restrictions. This may involve substituting ingredients, reducing sodium or sugar content, or avoiding certain foods altogether. Working with a registered dietitian can help identify suitable substitutions and create meal plans that meet individual dietary needs.

Consider Texture Modifications

Some seniors may have difficulty chewing or swallowing, which can make it challenging to eat certain foods. In these cases, it may be necessary to modify the texture of foods to make them easier to consume. This could involve pureeing fruits and vegetables, cutting meats into smaller pieces, or incorporating soft foods like yogurt or smoothies into the meal plan. Texture modifications can help seniors maintain a balanced diet while ensuring that they can safely eat and enjoy their meals.

Plan Ahead and Batch Cook

One of the key strategies for successful meal planning for seniors is to plan ahead and batch cook.

By preparing meals in advance and portioning them out into individual servings, seniors can ensure that they have healthy, nutritious meals readily available. This can help prevent reliance on convenience foods or takeout options, which are often high in sodium, sugar, and unhealthy fats.

Encourage Hydration

Staying hydrated is essential for seniors, as dehydration can lead to a range of health problems, including urinary tract infections, constipation, and cognitive decline. It is important to encourage seniors to drink plenty of fluids throughout the day, including water, herbal teas, and low-sugar beverages. Including hydrating foods like fruits and vegetables in meals can also contribute to overall fluid intake.

In conclusion, meal planning for seniors requires careful consideration of individual dietary needs and health conditions. By focusing on nutrient-rich foods, balanced meals, and adaptations for dietary restrictions, seniors can maintain a healthy and enjoyable diet that supports their overall well-being. Consulting with a healthcare provider or registered dietitian can provide valuable guidance and support in creating meal plans that meet the unique needs of seniors.

Incorporating more fruits and vegetables into your diet is essential for maintaining overall health and well-being. These nutrient-dense foods are rich in vitamins, minerals, antioxidants, and fiber, all of which are crucial for supporting various bodily functions and reducing the risk of chronic diseases. However, many individuals struggle to consume an adequate amount of fruits and vegetables on a daily basis. In this chapter, we will explore some creative and practical ideas for adding more fruits and vegetables to your diet, as well as the numerous health benefits they provide.

Ideas for Adding More Fruits and Vegetables to Your Diet:

Start your day with a fruit smoothie: Blend together a variety of fruits such as berries, bananas, and mangoes with some leafy greens like spinach or kale for a delicious and nutritious breakfast option.

You can also add some Greek yogurt or nut butter for extra protein and creaminess.

Snack on fresh fruits and vegetables: Keep a bowl of fresh fruit on your kitchen counter or cut up some veggies like carrots, bell peppers, and cucumber to have on hand for a quick and easy snack. Pair them with hummus, guacamole, or Greek yogurt dip for added flavor.

Add fruits and vegetables to your meals: Incorporate fruits into your salads, oatmeal, or yogurt for a pop of color and sweetness.

 Mix vegetables into your stir-fries, soups, pasta dishes, and casseroles to increase their nutrient content and fiber.

Experiment with different cooking methods: Roasting, grilling, steaming, or sautéing fruits and vegetables can enhance their natural flavors and textures. Try grilling peaches or pineapple for a sweet and smoky twist, or roasting Brussels sprouts with balsamic vinegar for a caramelized finish.

Substitute fruits and vegetables for processed snacks: Instead of reaching for a bag of chips or cookies, opt for sliced apples with almond butter, air-popped popcorn with nutritional yeast, or veggie sticks with salsa for a healthier and more satisfying snack.

Health Benefits of Fruits and Vegetables:

Rich in vitamins and minerals: Fruits and vegetables are excellent sources of essential vitamins and minerals that are necessary for various bodily functions, such as vitamin C for immune support, vitamin A for vision health, and potassium for heart health.

High in antioxidants: Antioxidants found in fruits and vegetables help protect cells from damage caused by free radicals, which can contribute to aging and chronic diseases. Berries, leafy greens, and citrus fruits are particularly rich in antioxidants.

Fiber-rich: Fruits and vegetables are high in dietary fiber, which helps promote digestive health, regulate blood sugar levels, and reduce the risk of cardiovascular disease.

Fiber also helps you feel full and satisfied, making it easier to maintain a healthy weight. Low in calories and fat: Most fruits and vegetables are low in calories and fat, making them ideal for weight management and overall health. They are also naturally cholesterol-free and sodium-free, making them heart-healthy options.

Supports hydration: Fruits and vegetables have high water content, which helps keep you hydrated and aids in digestion. Staying hydrated is crucial for maintaining energy levels, cognitive function, and overall well-being.

Incorporating more fruits and vegetables into your diet is a simple and effective way to improve your health and well-being.

By incorporating these nutrient-dense foods into your meals and snacks, you can reap the numerous health benefits they provide, from supporting immune function and reducing inflammation to promoting heart health and weight management.

 Experiment with different fruits and vegetables, cooking methods, and recipes to discover new and delicious ways to incorporate these powerhouse foods into your daily routine. By making fruits and vegetables a priority in your diet, you can nourish your body from the inside out and enjoy a lifetime of good health.

Chapter 5: Eating Well on a Budget

As we age, it becomes increasingly important to prioritize our health and well-being. One key aspect of maintaining good health is eating a nutritious diet. However, with limited income during retirement, sticking to a budget can be a challenge. Fortunately, there are several practical strategies that seniors can implement to eat healthy while still being mindful of their finances.

Plan Ahead One of the most effective ways to save money on groceries is to plan your meals in advance. Take some time each week to create a meal plan based on what you already have in your pantry and what is on sale at your local grocery store.

By making a shopping list and sticking to it, you can avoid impulse purchases and ensure that you only buy the items you need.

Buying items in bulk can be a cost-effective way to stock up on pantry staples such as rice, pasta, and canned goods. Look for sales on non-perishable items and buy in larger quantities to save money in the long run. You can also consider purchasing a membership to a warehouse club, where you can buy items in bulk at a discounted price.

Shop Seasonally Fruits and vegetables that are in season are often cheaper and more flavorful than those that are out of season. Visit your local farmers' market or look for sales at your grocery store to take advantage of seasonal produce.

You can also consider buying frozen or canned fruits and vegetables, which are often more affordable and have a longer shelf life.

Eating out can be expensive, so try to cook at home as much as possible. Not only is homemade food generally healthier, but it is also more budget-friendly. Look for simple recipes that use affordable ingredients and consider cooking in batches to save time and money. You can also try meal prepping, where you prepare several meals in advance and store them in the freezer for later use.

Use Coupons and Discounts Take advantage of coupons, sales, and discounts to save money on groceries. Many grocery stores offer loyalty programs that give you access to exclusive deals and discounts.

You can also look for coupons online or in your local newspaper.
 Additionally, consider shopping at discount stores or using senior discounts to save even more money on your grocery bill.

Avoid Wasting Food Food waste can be a significant drain on your budget, so try to avoid throwing away uneaten food. Make an effort to use up leftovers, repurpose ingredients, and freeze perishable items before they go bad. You can also consider composting food scraps to reduce waste and improve your environmental footprint.

Choose Affordable Proteins Protein is an essential component of a healthy diet, but it can also be expensive. Look for affordable sources of protein such as beans, lentils, eggs, and canned tuna. You can also consider buying cheaper cuts of meat or purchasing meat in bulk to save money.

Plant-based proteins, such as tofu and tempeh, are also affordable options that can help you meet your protein needs without breaking the bank.

By following these practical tips, seniors can eat well on a budget and prioritize their health without overspending. With a little planning and creativity, you can enjoy nutritious and delicious meals while still being mindful of your finances.

Chapter 6: Cooking for One or Two

When it comes to cooking for smaller households, there are unique challenges that may arise. Whether you are cooking for yourself or just one other person, it can be difficult to find recipes that are both delicious and practical. In this chapter, we will discuss tips for preparing meals for smaller households, including recipe ideas and portion control.

Tips for Preparing Meals for Smaller Households

Invest in quality kitchen tools: Investing in quality kitchen tools can make cooking for one or two much easier. Consider purchasing smaller-sized pots and pans, a mini food processor, and other tools that are designed for smaller portions.

This will help you avoid wasting ingredients and make meal preparation more efficient.

Plan ahead: Planning your meals in advance can help you avoid waste and ensure that you have everything you need on hand. Take some time each week to plan out your meals, make a shopping list, and prep ingredients in advance. This will save you time and stress during the week.

Embrace leftovers: Leftovers can be a lifesaver when cooking for one or two. Cook large batches of your favorite meals and freeze individual portions for later. You can also repurpose leftovers into new dishes to keep things interesting.

Get creative with ingredients: When cooking for one or two, it can be challenging to use up all of your ingredients before they go bad.

Get creative with your ingredients by using them in multiple dishes or finding new ways to incorporate them into your meals. For example, leftover vegetables can be used in a stir-fry or soup, and extra herbs can be turned into a pesto or sauce.

Focus on balance: When cooking for smaller households, it can be easy to fall into the trap of eating the same meals over and over again. Focus on creating balanced meals that include protein, vegetables, and whole grains to ensure you are getting all of the nutrients you need.

Recipe Ideas

Sheet Pan Chicken and Vegetables: This easy one-pan meal is perfect for smaller households.

Simply toss chicken breasts, your favorite vegetables, and seasonings on a sheet pan and bake until cooked through. Serve with a side of rice or quinoa for a complete meal.

Pasta Primavera: This light and fresh pasta dish is perfect for spring and summer. Cook your favorite pasta according to package instructions and toss with sautéed vegetables, olive oil, garlic, and Parmesan cheese. Serve with a side salad for a complete meal.

Mini Turkey Meatloaves: These mini meatloaves are a fun twist on a classic comfort food. Mix ground turkey with breadcrumbs, egg, and seasonings, then form into individual loaves and bake until cooked through. Serve with mashed potatoes and steamed green beans for a cozy meal.

Portion Control

Portion control is important when cooking for smaller households to avoid overeating and wasting food. Here are some tips for portion control:

Use smaller plates: Using smaller plates can help you visually control your portion sizes. Opt for salad plates instead of dinner plates to help you avoid overeating.

Measure ingredients: When cooking, it can be easy to eyeball portion sizes and end up with more food than you need. Use measuring cups and spoons to accurately portion out ingredients and avoid waste.

Pack leftovers: If you have leftovers from a meal, pack them up in individual portions and store them in the fridge or freezer for later.

 This will help you avoid overeating and make meal planning easier.

By following these tips for preparing meals for smaller households, including recipe ideas and portion control, you can create delicious and practical meals for yourself or just one other person. Experiment with different recipes, get creative with your ingredients, and focus on balance to ensure you are getting all of the nutrients you need. Happy cooking!

Chapter 7: Dining Out as a Senior

Eating out at restaurants can be a fun and enjoyable experience, but for seniors, it is important to make healthy choices to maintain overall well-being and health. Navigating restaurant menus can be overwhelming with so many tempting options, but with the right guidance, seniors can make informed decisions that support their health goals. In this chapter, we will explore tips and strategies for making healthy choices when dining out as a senior.

Guidance on Making Healthy Choices

When dining out as a senior, it is important to prioritize nutrient-dense foods that provide essential vitamins and minerals without excessive calories, sodium, or unhealthy fats.

Here are some tips to help you make healthy choices when eating out:

Choose lean protein sources: Opt for grilled chicken, fish, or lean cuts of meat to get your protein fix without the added saturated fat. Plant-based protein options like beans, lentils, and tofu are also great choices for seniors looking to reduce their meat consumption.

Load up on vegetables: Make vegetables the star of your meal by choosing dishes that are packed with colorful and nutrient-rich veggies. Steamed, sautéed, or roasted vegetables are great side dish options that can help you fill up without adding extra calories.

Watch your portion sizes: Many restaurants serve oversized portions that can contribute to overeating and weight gain. To avoid overeating, consider sharing a meal with a friend or asking for a half portion or to-go box to save some of your meal for later.

Limit added sugars and refined carbs: Be mindful of dishes that are high in added sugars and refined carbohydrates like white bread, pasta, and desserts. Opt for whole grain options when available and choose unsweetened beverages to cut down on unnecessary sugars.

Be cautious of hidden fats: Keep an eye out for dishes that are high in unhealthy fats like trans fats and saturated fats. Avoid fried foods and dishes that are heavy in creamy sauces, and instead, choose grilled or baked options that are lower in fat.

Navigating Restaurant Menus

Navigating restaurant menus can be overwhelming, especially with so many tempting options that may not always align with your health goals. Here are some tips to help you make informed decisions when faced with a menu full of delicious choices:

Plan ahead: Before going out to eat, take some time to look at the menu online or call ahead to inquire about healthy options. Knowing what to expect can help you make a more informed decision when it comes time to order.

Look for keywords: Pay attention to words on the menu that can give you clues about how a dish is prepared.

Opt for items that are grilled, steamed, baked, or roasted, and avoid dishes that are fried, breaded, or smothered in creamy sauces.

Ask for modifications: Don't be afraid to ask for modifications to suit your dietary needs. Restaurants are often willing to accommodate special requests like swapping out sides for healthier options, dressing on the side, or skipping certain ingredients.

Choose wisely: Instead of automatically going for your favorite dish, take the time to explore the menu and consider healthier alternatives. Look for dishes that are packed with vegetables, lean proteins, and whole grains to ensure a balanced meal.

Practice portion control: Be mindful of portion sizes and avoid the temptation to overindulge.
Consider ordering an appetizer or splitting a main dish with a friend to help control your portion sizes and prevent overeating.

By following these tips and strategies, seniors can make healthy choices when dining out and enjoy delicious meals without compromising their health goals. With a little planning and mindfulness, eating out can be a rewarding experience that supports overall well-being and longevity.

Chapter 8: Overcoming Common Challenges

Maintaining a healthy diet is essential for overall well-being, but it can be difficult to achieve for some individuals facing common obstacles such as limited mobility or difficulty chewing. However, with the right strategies in place, it is possible to overcome these challenges and continue to eat healthily. In this chapter, we will explore various techniques and accommodations that can help individuals address these common obstacles and maintain a nutritious diet.

Limited Mobility

Limited mobility can make it challenging to prepare meals, access healthy food options, and even eat comfortably.

However, there are several strategies that can help individuals overcome these challenges and continue to eat healthily.

Meal delivery services: One way to overcome the challenge of limited mobility is to utilize meal delivery services that offer nutritious, pre-prepared meals. These services can provide individuals with a variety of healthy options that are delivered directly to their door, making it easier to maintain a balanced diet.

Meal planning and preparation: For individuals who are able to prepare their own meals with limited mobility, meal planning and preparation can help streamline the process. By planning out meals in advance and prepping ingredients ahead of time, individuals can reduce the time and effort required to cook healthy meals.

Kitchen modifications: Making small modifications to the kitchen can also help individuals with limited mobility cook and prepare meals more easily. This may include installing grab bars, lowering countertops, or using adaptive kitchen tools to make cooking more accessible.

Family and caregiver support: For individuals with limited mobility, enlisting the help of family members or caregivers can make a significant difference in maintaining a healthy diet. By having assistance with meal preparation and grocery shopping, individuals can ensure they are getting the nutrition they need.

Difficulty Chewing

Difficulty chewing can make it challenging to consume certain types of foods, which can limit the variety of nutrients individuals are able to obtain from their diet.
However, there are strategies that can help individuals with difficulty chewing still eat a nutritious diet.

Texture modifications: One way to address difficulty chewing is to modify the texture of foods to make them easier to eat. This may include pureeing or mashing foods, or choosing soft, easily chewable options such as cooked vegetables or tender meats.

Nutrient-dense foods: For individuals with difficulty chewing, it is important to focus on consuming nutrient-dense foods that are easy to eat.

This may include smoothies, soups, and other blended options that can provide a variety of nutrients without requiring extensive chewing.

Dental consultation: Individuals experiencing difficulty chewing should consider consulting with a dentist or oral health specialist to address any underlying issues that may be contributing to the problem. By addressing dental concerns, individuals may find it easier to eat a wider variety of foods.

Dietary supplements: In some cases, individuals with difficulty chewing may benefit from incorporating dietary supplements into their routine to ensure they are receiving all the necessary nutrients.

It is important to consult with a healthcare provider before adding any supplements to the diet.

By implementing these strategies and accommodations, individuals with limited mobility or difficulty chewing can overcome common obstacles to healthy eating and continue to maintain a balanced, nutritious diet. With a focus on finding creative solutions and seeking support when needed, individuals can ensure they are getting the nutrients they need for optimal health and well-being.

Chapter 9: Staying Hydrated

As we age, our bodies experience changes that can affect our hydration levels. It becomes increasingly important for seniors to pay attention to their fluid intake in order to maintain good health and well-being. In this chapter, we will explore the importance of staying hydrated as a senior and provide tips on how to ensure you are getting enough fluids throughout the day.

The Importance of Staying Hydrated

Water is essential for our bodies to function properly. It helps regulate body temperature, lubricate joints, transport nutrients, and remove waste. Dehydration can lead to a variety of health issues, including urinary tract infections, constipation, kidney stones, and even confusion or delirium.

As we age, our bodies may not signal thirst as effectively, which can lead to decreased fluid intake. Additionally, certain medications or health conditions can increase the risk of dehydration. It is crucial for seniors to be proactive about staying hydrated to prevent these negative consequences.

Tips for Getting Enough Fluids Throughout the Day

Drink Plenty of Water: The best way to stay hydrated is to drink plenty of water throughout the day. Aim for at least 8-10 cups of water daily, or more if you are physically active or live in a hot climate. Keep a water bottle with you at all times as a reminder to drink.

Eat Hydrating Foods: Many fruits and vegetables have high water content and can help contribute to your overall fluid intake. Watermelon, cucumbers, oranges, and tomatoes are all excellent choices. Soups and broths can also be a good source of hydration.

Monitor Your Urine: One simple way to gauge your hydration status is to pay attention to the color of your urine. Pale yellow or straw-colored urine indicates that you are well-hydrated, while darker urine may be a sign that you need to drink more water.

Set Reminders: As we age, it can be easy to forget to drink enough water throughout the day. Set reminders on your phone or use a timer to prompt yourself to take a sip of water regularly.

Limit Diuretics: Some beverages, such as caffeinated or alcoholic drinks, can have a diuretic effect and increase fluid loss. Limit your intake of these beverages and opt for water or decaffeinated options instead.

Stay Cool: In hot weather, it is especially important to stay hydrated to prevent dehydration and heat-related illnesses. Drink extra water and avoid excessive exertion during the hottest parts of the day.

Talk to Your Doctor: If you have a medical condition that affects your hydration levels, or if you are taking medications that can impact fluid balance, talk to your doctor about how to stay hydrated safely.

Remember, staying hydrated is a crucial part of maintaining good health as a senior.

By following these tips and being proactive about your fluid intake, you can help prevent dehydration and its associated complications. Prioritize your hydration and make it a priority in your daily routine.

Maintaining a healthy diet long-term and making lasting changes to eating habits can be a challenging but rewarding endeavor. By following the advice outlined in this chapter, you can create a sustainable healthy eating plan that will not only improve your overall health and well-being but also provide you with the energy and vitality needed to live your best life.

Advice on how to maintain a healthy diet long-term and make lasting changes to eating habits:

Focus on whole, nutrient-dense foods: When creating a healthy eating plan, it is essential to focus on consuming whole,

nutrient-dense foods such as fruits, vegetables, whole grains, lean proteins, and healthy fats.
These foods are rich in essential nutrients that your body needs to function optimally and can help you feel full and satisfied.

Avoid processed and refined foods: Processed and refined foods are often high in unhealthy fats, sugars, and empty calories, which can contribute to weight gain and increase your risk of chronic diseases. Avoiding these foods and opting for whole, minimally processed alternatives can help you maintain a healthy diet long-term.

Practice portion control: Overeating can lead to weight gain and other health issues, so it is essential to practice portion control when planning your meals.

Pay attention to your hunger and fullness cues, and aim to eat until you are satisfied, not overly full.

Stay hydrated: Drinking an adequate amount of water each day is essential for maintaining optimal health and supporting your body's various functions. Aim to drink at least eight 8-ounce glasses of water daily, and consider adding hydrating foods such as fruits and vegetables to your meals.

Plan ahead: Planning your meals and snacks in advance can help you make healthy choices and avoid impulse eating. Take the time to create a weekly meal plan and grocery list, and consider meal prepping to save time and ensure that healthy options are readily available.

Practice mindful eating: Mindful eating involves paying attention to your food choices, eating slowly, and savoring each bite. By practicing mindful eating, you can better tune into your body's hunger and fullness cues, leading to improved digestion and better overall health.

Seek support: Making lasting changes to your eating habits can be challenging, so it is essential to seek support from friends, family, or a healthcare professional. Consider enlisting the help of a registered dietitian or nutritionist to create a personalized eating plan that meets your individual needs and goals.

Conclusion and Next Steps:

Creating a sustainable healthy eating plan is a journey that requires dedication, patience, and a willingness to make positive changes. By following the advice outlined in this chapter and seeking support when needed, you can develop healthy eating habits that will benefit you for years to come. Remember that small, consistent changes over time can lead to significant improvements in your health and well-being. Stay committed to your goals, be kind to yourself, and enjoy the process of nourishing your body with nutritious foods. Your future self will thank you for it.

Suggested Food Guide

A healthy food guide for seniors should include a variety of nutrient-rich foods that support overall health and well-being. Here are some key components to include:

1. Fruits and Vegetables: Encourage seniors to incorporate a colorful array of fruits and vegetables into their diet. These provide essential vitamins, minerals, antioxidants, and fiber. Aim for a variety of types and colors to ensure a diverse range of nutrients.
2. Whole Grains: Opt for whole grains like brown rice, quinoa, whole wheat bread, and oatmeal over refined grains. Whole grains provide fiber, vitamins, and minerals, and they help support digestive health and regulate blood sugar levels.

3. Lean Proteins: Include sources of lean protein such as poultry, fish, beans, lentils, tofu, and low-fat dairy products. Protein is important for maintaining

4. muscle mass, bone health, and overall strength.

5. Healthy Fats: Incorporate sources of healthy fats, such as avocados, nuts, seeds, and olive oil. These fats are essential for brain health, heart health, and absorption of fat-soluble vitamins.

6. Low-Fat Dairy or Dairy Alternatives: Choose low-fat or non-fat dairy products like milk, yogurt, and cheese, or opt for dairy alternatives like fortified soy or almond milk.

7. Hydration: Encourage seniors to stay hydrated by drinking plenty of water throughout the day. Offer water as the main beverage choice and limit sugary drinks and excessive caffeine.

8. Limit Processed Foods and Sugary
   Snacks: Encourage seniors to minimize
   intake of processed foods, sugary
   snacks, and high-sodium foods.
   Instead, focus on whole, minimally
   processed foods to support overall
   health.
9. Portion Control: Encourage portion
   control to prevent overeating and
   maintain a healthy weight. Use smaller
   plates and bowls to help manage
   portion sizes.
10.   Mindful Eating: Encourage seniors to
   practice mindful eating by paying
   attention to hunger and fullness cues,
   savoring each bite, and eating slowly.

11. Variety and Moderation: Emphasize the importance of variety and moderation in the diet. Encourage seniors to enjoy a wide range of foods in moderation to ensure they receive a balance of nutrients.

By following these guidelines, seniors can enjoy a nutritious and well-balanced diet that supports their overall health and well-being.

Here's a sample healthy menu for seniors that incorporates a variety of nutrient-rich foods:

Breakfast:

- Oatmeal topped with fresh berries and a sprinkle of chopped nuts
- Scrambled eggs with spinach and tomatoes
- Whole grain toast with avocado slices
- Low-fat Greek yogurt with a drizzle of honey

Lunch:

- Grilled chicken salad with mixed greens, cherry tomatoes, cucumbers, and balsamic vinaigrette
- Quinoa and vegetable stir-fry with tofu or shrimp
- Whole grain wrap filled with hummus, sliced turkey, lettuce, and shredded carrots
- Lentil soup with a side of whole grain crackers

Dinner:

- Baked salmon with roasted sweet potatoes and steamed broccoli
- Turkey meatballs with whole wheat pasta and marinara sauce
- Stir-fried tofu and mixed vegetables served over brown rice
- Grilled lean steak with roasted Brussels sprouts and quinoa pilaf

Snacks:

- Apple slices with almond butter
- Carrot sticks with hummus
- Greek yogurt with a sprinkle of granola
- Air-popped popcorn
- A handful of mixed nuts and dried fruit

Beverages:

- Water with lemon or cucumber slices
- Herbal tea
- Low-fat milk or fortified plant-based milk

This menu provides a balance of lean proteins, whole grains, fruits, vegetables, and healthy fats to support overall health and well-being in seniors. Adjust portion sizes as needed based on individual dietary needs and preferences. Additionally, consider any specific dietary restrictions or health conditions when planning meals.

NOTES

NOTES

NOTES

THANK YOU FOR YOUR SUPPORT

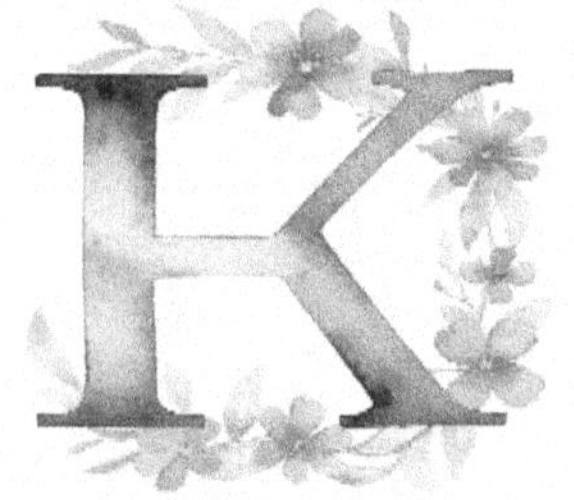